I0415869

Contents

The employer is required to post a copy of this report for 30 days at or near the workplace(s) of affected employees. The employer must take steps to ensure that the posted report is not altered, defaced, or covered by other material.

The cover photo is a close-up image of sorbent tubes, which are used by the HHE Program to measure airborne exposures. This photo is an artistic representation that may not be related to this Health Hazard Evaluation.

Highlights of this Evaluation

The Health Hazard Evaluation Program received a request from an outpatient pharmacy. The employer was concerned about employee exposures to pharmaceutical dust.

What We Did

- We did exposure sampling at the pharmacy in April 2011. We returned in April 2012 to do more sampling.

- We measured particle levels over time at different processes. We did this to determine if pharmaceutical dust was released into the air.

- We sampled the air for dust. These air samples were weighed to determine the amount of dust in the air. They were also analyzed for lactose (common inactive filler in tablets) and active pharmaceutical ingredients.

- We sampled surfaces for lactose to look for possible pharmaceutical contamination throughout the pharmacy.

What We Found

- One employee was exposed to lisinopril on two workdays at levels near or above the manufacturer's exposure limit.

- Dust was released into the air when automatic dispensing machine canisters were cleaned with compressed air. Filling canisters with tablets produced lower levels of dust in the air.

> Work activities in the outpatient pharmacy generated dusts that exposed employees to pharmaceutical ingredients. One employee had personal air concentrations of lisinopril near or above the manufacturer's exposure limit. We recommend doing dust-generating tasks under a local exhaust hood and using a vacuum with high-efficiency particulate air filtration to clean canisters.

- After employees used compressed air to clean canisters, more than an hour passed before the small particles produced were no longer in the air.

- We found lactose and active pharmaceutical ingredients in the dust in the air. Lactose was found on surfaces throughout the pharmacy. This suggests that some dust in air and on surfaces was from pharmaceuticals.

- Some employees wore nitrile gloves when handling pharmaceuticals. Employees did not wear protective clothing or safety glasses.

What the Employer Can Do

- Develop a list of pharmaceuticals that are dusty and gather exposure guidelines and toxicity data for those pharmaceuticals. Use this information to guide future exposure assessments and determine how these pharmaceuticals should be handled.

- Install a partially-enclosed local exhaust hood for cleaning and filling canisters with tablets or doing other tasks that could send pharmaceutical dust into the air.

What the Employer Can Do (continued)

- Continue to use the vacuum daily to clean the Optifill machine. Make sure the vacuum contains a high efficiency particulate air filter. Change the filter routinely according to the manufacturer's guidelines.

- Use the vacuum with a long narrow nozzle to clean canisters. Stop using compressed air for this task.

- Provide safety glasses and protective clothing to employees who do tasks outside the hood that could send pharmaceutical dust into the air.

- Train employees on the need to wear nitrile gloves when handling pharmaceuticals.

- Clean work surfaces with alcohol wipes before breaks and at the end of the workday.

- Create a health and safety committee. This committee should include employee and employer representatives who meet regularly to address health and safety concerns.

What Employees Can Do

- Follow the procedures for using and maintaining the local exhaust hood.

- Wear nitrile gloves when handling pharmaceuticals.

- Wash your hands before you eat, drink, or use tobacco products.

- Tell your supervisor about workplace health or safety concerns you have.

- Become active in the health and safety committee.

Mention of any company or product does not constitute endorsement by NIOSH. In addition, citations to websites external to NIOSH do not constitute NIOSH endorsement of the sponsoring organizations or their programs or products. Furthermore, NIOSH is not responsible for the content of these websites. All web addresses referenced in this document were accessible as of the publication date of this report.

Abbreviations

°C	Degrees Celsius
$\mu g/cm^2$	Micrograms per square centimeter
$\mu g/m^3$	Micrograms per cubic meter
μm	Micrometer
API	Active pharmaceutical ingredient
BVNA	Bureau Veritas North America, Inc.
CFR	Code of Federal Regulations
HCTZ	Hydrochlorothiazide
HEPA	High-efficiency particulate air
HHPC	Handheld airborne particle counter
IOM	Institute of Occupational Medicine
Lpm	Liters per minute
MDC	Minimum detectable concentration
mL	Milliliter
mm	Millimeter
mM	Millimolar
MQC	Minimum quantifiable concentration
n	Number of samples
NA	Not applicable
NAICS	North American Industry Classification System
ND	Not detected
NIOSH	National Institute for Occupational Safety and Health
No.	Number
OEL	Occupational exposure limit
p/L	Particles per liter
PTFE	Polytetrafluoroethylene
TWA	Time-weighted average

Introduction

The Health Hazard Evaluation Program received a request from managers at an outpatient pharmacy in Ohio. The request concerned potential employee exposures to pharmaceutical dust. We evaluated exposures at the pharmacy in April 2011 and April 2012.

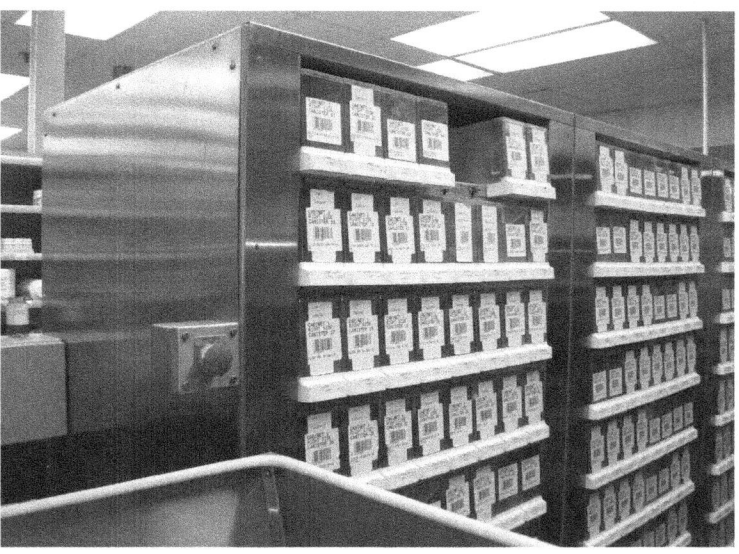

Figure 1. Optifill machine.

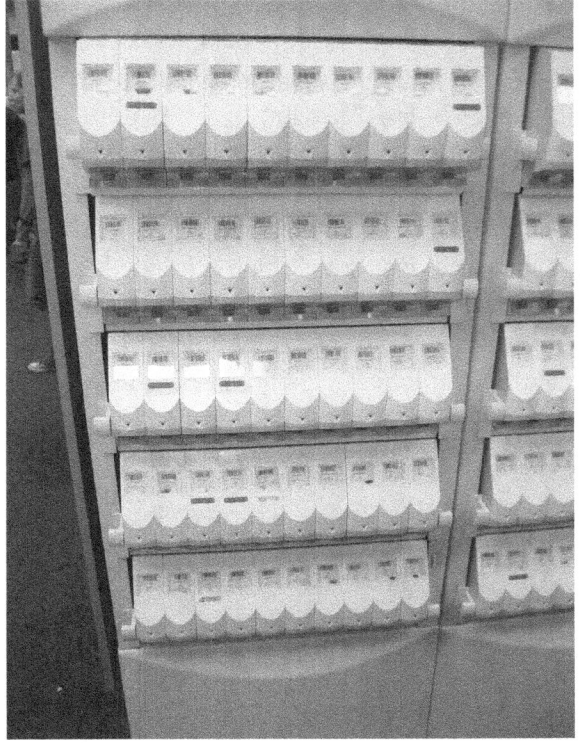

Figure 2. PharmAssist machine.

Twenty or more employees worked at the pharmacy, which operated a single shift 6 days per week (Monday through Saturday). The pharmacy filled 7,000 to 8,000 prescriptions per week primarily using automatic dispensing machines. An Optifill® II-Plus machine (Figure 1, AmerisourceBergen®, Valley Forge, Pennsylvania) was used for most refills and a PharmAssist® machine (Figure 2, Innovation, Johnson City, New York) was used for filling most initial prescriptions. On occasion, some technicians used a desktop counter (model no. KL15df, KirbyLester, Lake Forest, Illinois) to fill prescriptions. All these machines used gravity to dispense pharmaceutical tablets and capsules. One pharmacy technician hand filled prescriptions for controlled substances (schedule II–V) in a dedicated area. Some prescriptions did not require any counting as they came prepackaged from the manufacturer as a unit dose or the usual prescribed dose. All prescriptions were verified by pharmacists.

The Optifill machine was maintained by two pharmacy technicians. Maintenance activities included refilling canisters; using compressed air to clean canisters; and cleaning the inside of the Optifill machine with a 3M field service vacuum (3M, St. Paul, Minnesota), isopropyl alcohol wipes, and stainless steel cleaner. Several pharmacy technicians shared the maintenance of the PharmAssist machine. Maintenance included refilling canisters and using compressed air to clean canisters. Canisters required cleaning if they were extremely dusty or stopped functioning properly, usually due to dust accumulation.

Methods

The purpose of this evaluation was to (1) determine if and during which activities dust was released into the air, (2) measure the concentration of the airborne dust, (3) quantify specific active pharmaceutical agents (APIs) and other pharmaceutical ingredients in the airborne dust, and (4) determine the extent of surface contamination with pharmaceutical ingredients.

Air Sampling

The air sampling methods used during visit 1 (April 2011) are summarized in Table 1. Seven total dust air samples were collected in the personal breathing zones of employees with (n = 4) and without (n = 3) an inline Personal DataRAM aerosol monitor (Thermo, Smyrna, Georgia), and six total dust air samples were collected at fixed locations in the pharmacy with (n = 2) and without (n = 4) an inline DustTrak aerosol monitor (TSI®, St. Paul, Minnesota). When sampling with the personal DataRAM, air was drawn through the inlet of Tygon® tubing positioned in the employee's breathing zone. The primary purpose of visit 1 was to identify the processes that produced the most dust so we could follow up with more detailed sampling during visit 2 (April 2012).

The air and surface sampling methods used during visit 2 are summarized in Table 2. Over a period of three days, 27 inhalable dust air samples were collected. Nine personal air samples were collected, including two sets of side-by-side air samples worn on opposite shoulders on two separate days by the same employee. Side-by-side sampling was done to allow us to quantify more than one API in an employee's breathing zone and to compare air concentrations measured on one side of the body to the other side of the body. Another 18 area air samples were collected at fixed locations throughout the pharmacy. Total and inhalable dust air samples are intended to measure airborne dust that could be inhaled and deposited anywhere in the respiratory system (including the nose and mouth) [Kenny 1997, ACGIH 2012]. However, compared to an inhalable dust sample, a total dust sample (in closed-face configuration) has been shown to undersample particles greater than 30 micrometers (µm) in aerodynamic diameter because of its smaller inlet [Kenny 1997]. This issue prompted the sole use of inhalable dust samples for visit 2.

Table 1. Summary of the air sampling methods used during visit 1

Sampling media/ equipment	Flow rate (Lpm)	Analytes	Method	No. of personal samples	No. of area samples
Tared 37-mm PTFE filter, closed face cassette (n = 7)	4	Total dust (by mass)	NIOSH Method 0500*	3	4
Tared 37-mm PTFE filter, Personal DataRAM (n = 4) aerosol monitor	2.2	Total dust (in real time)	NA	4	0
		Total dust (by mass)	NIOSH Method 0500*	4	0
Tared 37-mm PTFE filter, DustTrak™ DRX aerosol monitor (n = 2)	3	Total dust (in real time)	NA	NA	2
		Total dust (by mass)	NIOSH Method 0500*	NA	2
HHPC-6 optical particle counter	NA	Particle count (in real time)	NA	NA	NA

HHPC = handheld airborne particle counter

Lpm = liters per minute

mm = millimeter

NA = not applicable

NIOSH = National Institute for Occupational Safety and Health

PTFE = polytetrafluoroethylene

*NIOSH Manual of Analytical Methods [NIOSH 2010]

Table 2. Summary of the air and surface sampling methods used during visit 2

Sampling media/ equipment	Flow rate (Lpm)	Analytes	Method	No. of personal samples	No. of area samples
Air sampling					
Tared 25-mm PTFE filter, IOM sampler (n = 27)	2	Inhalable dust (by mass)	NIOSH Method 0600*	9	18
		Lactose	BVNA internal method†	7	15
		Lisinopril	BVNA internal method†	3	3
		HCTZ	BVNA internal method†	3	0
		Loratadine	BVNA internal method†	1	0
		Hydrocodone bitartrate	BVNA internal method†	0	2
		Oxycodone	BVNA internal method†	0	2
		Codeine	BVNA internal method†	0	2
		Levothyroxine	BVNA internal method†	1	0
		Atenolol	BVNA internal method†	0	1
HHPC-6 optical particle counter	NA	Particle count (in real time)	NA	NA	NA
Surface sampling					
Alpha Texwipe pre-wetted with deionized water	NA	Lactose	BVNA internal method†	NA	18

BVNA = Bureau Veritas North America

HCTZ = hydrochlorothiazide

IOM = Institute of Medicine

*NIOSH Manual of Analytical Methods [NIOSH 2010]

†More information on the BVNA analytical methods is provided in Appendix A.

During both visits, we followed some of the employees throughout their workday and held HHPC-6 real-time particle counters near their breathing zones to identify dusty tasks (i.e., peaks in particle concentration) (Figure 3). We also recorded the types of tablets handled so that we could later identify air samples collected during visit 2 (previously analyzed gravimetrically) to be further analyzed for lactose (a common inactive filler in tablets) and/or specific APIs (Table 2). Most of these air samples were analyzed for lactose, lisinopril, and HCTZ. Only a few of these air samples were analyzed for other APIs.

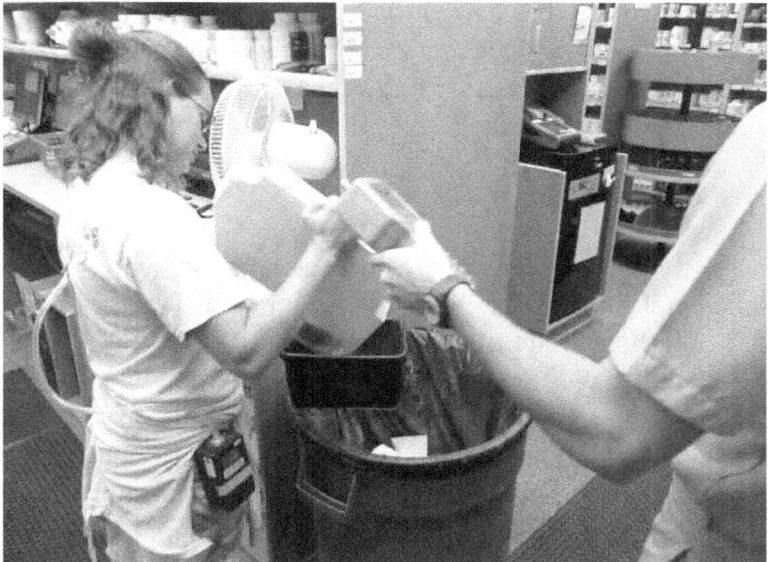

Figure 3. Using a real-time particle counter to measure particle concentration near the personal breathing zone of an employee cleaning a PharmAssist canister.

During visit 2, we sampled 18 surfaces for lactose contamination (Table 2). This was done to estimate the extent of pharmaceutical dust contamination throughout the pharmacy. Templates (10 centimeters by 10 centimeters) were placed on top of a surface. While wearing nitrile gloves, we wiped the area inside the template with a prewetted towelette in three different directions. For irregularly shaped surfaces, the investigator estimated approximate 100 square-centimeter areas and wiped the surface in a manner identical to that used for flat surfaces. Appendix A provides more information on the sampling and analytical methods.

Results

Airborne Pharmaceutical Dust

Real-Time Particle Concentrations

Results of the real-time particle measurements are in Figures B1–B6 of Appendix B. We used this information to decide which APIs to measure on the inhalable dust samples. The DustTrak data and some of the DataRAM and HHPC-6 data are not presented because they did not add to the information provided in Figures B1–B6. These figures show peaks in particle number and mass concentrations that were correlated with events involving specific APIs. Refilling canisters with uncoated tablets produced some airborne dust (Figures B4 and B6); however, the highest transient particle mass concentrations of total dust (up to 9,500 micrograms per cubic meter [$\mu g/m^3$]) and total particle number concentrations (up to 350,000 particles per liter [p/L]) were observed during the cleaning of canisters using compressed air (Figures B1 and B4). In most cases, these canisters housed uncoated tablets. After using compressed air, in some cases it took > 60 minutes for the number concentration of particles < 1 μm in aerodynamic diameter to return to the baseline concentration measured prior to the cleaning activity (Figures B2 and B5).

Particles < 1 μm in aerodynamic diameter were elevated (up to 45,000 p/L) during the cleaning of the Optifill machine using a vacuum (Figure B4). The vacuum was capable of delivering high-efficiency particulate air (HEPA) filtration; however, the vacuum contained a non-HEPA designated 3M type II filter designed for copier/printer toner ink and dust (product no. 78-8005-5350-1). The task-based personal air concentration of inhalable dust collected (over 33 minutes) from employee 23 performing this task was 2,000 μg/m³. The dust that was collected in this employee's breathing zone also contained lactose (5.2 μg/m³), but the other APIs (e.g., HCTZ and lisinopril) were not-detected (ND).

Air Concentrations of Total Dust during Visit 1

Tables 3 and 4 provide the personal and area air concentrations of total dust for visit 1. Figure 4 shows the locations of the area air samples for visit 1. The air concentrations in these and subsequent tables are presented as 8-hour time-weighted averages (TWAs) or longer duration TWAs if the sample time was > 480 minutes. We stopped sampling only after employees finished working with pharmaceuticals. Therefore, we assumed zero exposure for any unsampled time periods during an 8-hour work shift. The minimum detectable concentrations (MDCs) and minimum quantifiable concentrations (MQCs) provided in these and subsequent tables were calculated by dividing the analytical limits of detection and quantitation (mass units) for each analyte by the average volume of air that would have been sampled over an 8-hour period (unless otherwise noted). The MDCs and MQCs represent the smallest air concentrations that could have been detected (MDC) or quantified (MQC).

Four of the personal total dust air samples (Table 3) were collected using sample media in line with a personal DataRAM. Tygon tubing was connected to the DataRAM, and the inlet of the tubing was positioned in the personal breathing zone. According to guidelines from the DataRAM manufacturer, use of the Tygon tubing can result in > 50% loss of particles > 10 μm in aerodynamic diameter [Thermo 1995]. This could explain why most of the levels collected by these samples were ND. One of these samples (no. 133), however, collected 140 μg/m³ of total dust. The cleaning of a canister with compressed air was likely the main source of this dust. According to the real-time particle number concentrations measured during this task (Figure B3 in Appendix B), a large portion of this dust was < 3 μm in aerodynamic diameter. At this particle size, any losses from the Tygon tubing would be < 10% [Thermo 1995]. Nevertheless, the total dust concentrations obtained using sample media in line with a DataRAM likely underestimated the actual concentrations.

Table 3. Work-shift personal air concentrations of total dust for visit 1

Day	Employee ID	Process description	Sample no.*	Sample time (minutes)	TWA personal air concentration of total dust (µg/m³)†
1	11	PharmAssist and Optifill canister cleaning	14	280	410
	12	Manual counting, middle station	134	352	ND‡
	13	Optifill canister refill	135	289	ND‡
	14	Manual counting, station #1	15	400	ND
2	11	PharmAssist and Optifill canister refill and cleaning	133	444	(140)‡
	12	Packaging, end of line	12	487	(42)
	13	Optifill canister refill	131	457	ND‡
MDC					60
MQC					180

*Sample numbers are provided for referring to the figures in Appendix B.

†TWA over 8 hours. Assumed zero exposure during any unsampled periods. If sample time was > 480 minutes, then the TWA over that time period is provided. Values between the MDC and MQC are shown in parentheses to point out that there is more uncertainty associated with these values than with concentrations above the MQC.

‡Air in an employee's personal breathing zone was drawn through tubing into a personal DataRAM and then collected on sample media. The mass concentration measured by the sample media may underestimate the actual concentration because of particle losses in the tubing.

Table 4. Work-shift area air concentrations of total dust for visit 1

Sample duration	Day	Location description	Sample no.*	Sample time (minutes)	TWA area air concentration of total dust (µg/m³)†
Work shift (~8 hours)	1	Top of PharmAssist Pod B	19	395	(52)
	2	Top of PharmAssist Pod B	110	490	ND
		Workstation next to PharmAssist Pod A	13	385	ND
		Manual fill station #1	18	384	ND
	MDC				40
	MQC				140
> 30 hours	1 and 2	Shelf #1, next to Optifill machine	115	1864	(23)‡
		Shelf #2, west end, close to manual fill station #2	112	1860	(14)‡
	MDC				10§
	MQC				47§

*Sample numbers are provided for referring to the sample locations in Figure 4.

†TWA over 8 hours. Assumed zero exposure during any unsampled periods. If sample time was > 480 minutes, then the TWA over that time period is provided. Values between the MDC and MQC are shown in parentheses to point out that there is more uncertainty associated with these values than with concentrations above the MQC.

‡Collected using sample media in line with a DustTrak aerosol monitor.

§Calculated using average volume of air that was sampled over 1,860 minutes.

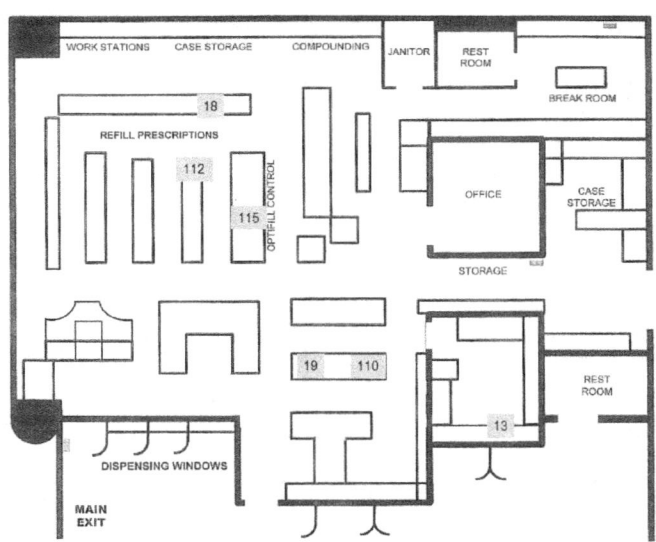

Figure 4. Area air sample locations during visit 1.

Air Concentrations of Inhalable Dust, Lactose, and Active Pharmaceutical Ingredients during Visit 2

Tables 5 and 6 provide the personal and area air concentrations of inhalable dust, lactose, lisinopril, and HCTZ (personal only) for visit 2. Figure 5 shows the locations of the area air samples for visit 2. The manufacturer's occupational exposure limits (OELs) for lisinopril and HCTZ [Bristol-Myers Squibb Company 2012a,b] are provided in Tables 5 and 6. The lower bound of the manufacturer's hazard control band for lisinopril [Bristol-Myers Squibb Company 2012b] was used for comparing employee exposures and is the most conservative way of establishing an OEL on the basis of a hazard control band. More information on control banding and OELs is provided in Appendix C.

Table 5. Work-shift personal air concentrations of inhalable dust, lactose, and select APIs during visit 2

| Day | Employee ID | Process description | Sample no.† | Sample time (minutes) | TWA personal air concentration (µg/m³)‡ | | | |
					Inhalable dust	Lactose	Lisinopril	HCTZ
1	21	Optifill canister refill and cleaning and manual counting*	223/25	350	Error§	5.3	0.96	(0.24)
			225/25	351	(130)	3.7	0.55	(0.17)
	22	Vault hand filling and canister cleaning	213	366	(400)	NA	NA	NA
			216	405	(350)	NA	NA	NA
2	21	Optifill canister refill and cleaning	230	341	ND	3.3	NA	NA
			231	285	ND	5.6	1.1	(0.20)
	24	Manual counting	23	162	(150)	1.7	NA	NA
MDC					100	0.003	0.1	0.1
MQC					320	0.0089	0.35	0.35
Manufacturer's OEL							1¶	100¶

*Optifill canister cleaning was done in the morning (~130 minutes), and manual counting was done in the afternoon (~220 minutes).

†Sample numbers are provided for referring to the figures in Appendix B. If more than one set of sample numbers is listed per process description, then side-by-side air sampling was performed.

‡TWA over 8 hours. Assumed zero exposure during any unsampled periods. If sample time was > 480 minutes, then the TWA over that time period is provided.

§A large piece of debris (not pharmaceutical) was collected by the sample media. This made gravimetric analysis unreliable.

¶According to safety data sheets [Bristol-Myers Squibb Company 2012a b]. The OEL for lisinopril is the lower bound of the hazard control band (1–10 µg/m³).

Table 6. Work-shift area air concentrations of inhalable dust, lactose and lisinopril during visit 2

Day	Location description	Sample no.*	Sample time (minutes)	TWA area air concentration (µg/m³)†		
				Inhalable dust	Lactose	Lisinopril
1	Captain's office to the left inside the door (6 feet high)	215	566	ND	0.98	ND
	Shelf #4 to the south of the Optifill machine	217	543	(118)	2.8	(0.27)
	Pharmacist checking station (6 feet high)	218	565	(120)	2.3	NA
	Just north of supervisor's desk behind the belt	221	553	(140)	5.4	NA
	Break room on top of fridge (5.5 feet)	229	552	ND	1.7	ND
	Optifill workstation top shelf (7 feet above fan)	236	550	(140)	46	NA
	North side of PharmAssist machine (5.5 feet high)	237	544	ND	3.3	(0.18)
	Below 40-59 cabinet to the east of the Optifill (3.5 feet high)	239	558	ND	2.3	NA
	Shelf to the south of vault work station (4 feet high)	240	569	ND	0.34	ND
2	South wall of the Pod A room (6 feet high)	21	521	ND	0.02	NA
	On fridge in break room (5.5 feet high)	27	507	ND	0.16	NA
	North end of the manual fill table, near the compressed air line	29	521	(110)	1.2	(0.24)
	Below the 40-59 cabinet to the east of the optifill machine (3.5 feet high)	210	495	(140)	0.33	ND
	Corner just east of the janitor's closet (5.5 feet high)	211	500	(230)	0.37	NA
	Above the pharmacist checking station, north end (5 feet high)	212	500	(160)	0.25	NA
	Vault corner shelf (6 feet high)	214	484	(160)	ND	NA
	Checking station	226	482	ND	ND	NA
	Manual fill station #2	232	517	ND	ND	NA
MDC				100	0.003	0.1
MQC				290	0.008	0.32

*Sample numbers are provided for referring to sample locations in Figure 5.

†TWA over the sampled time period.

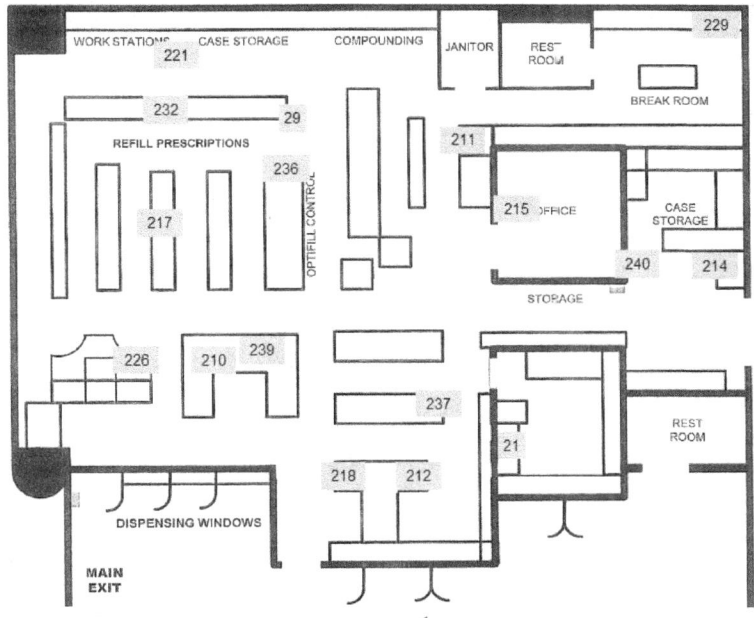

Figure 5. Area air sample locations during visit 2.

We compared the work-shift TWA personal air concentrations to published manufacturers' OELs (Table C1 in Appendix C). All HCTZ personal air concentrations were below the manufacturer's OEL. Employee 21 had personal air concentrations of lisinopril during two workdays that were near (0.96 µg/m³) or above (1.1 µg/m³) the manufacturer's OEL of 1 µg/m³. This employee refilled and cleaned Optifill canisters during both workdays. Employee 22, who cleaned canisters containing loratadine and levothyroxine (Figure B5 in Appendix B), had a personal air concentration of loratadine of 6.5 µg/m³ and a personal air concentration of levothyroxine of 0.0068 µg/m³. The levothyroxine concentration was below the manufacturer's OEL of < 1 µg/m³ [Pfizer 2011]. We were not able to find a published manufacturer's OEL for loratadine.

Area air concentrations of hydrocodone, oxycodone, codeine, and atenolol were ND (below their MDCs). The MDCs of hydrocodone, codeine, and atenolol were 0.10 µg/m³, and the MDC of oxycodone was 0.01 µg/m³. The MDCs of hydrocodone, codeine, and oxycodone were well below the manufacturers' OELs [GlaxoSmithKline 2006; Purdue Pharma 2008; Abbott Labs 2011]. We were not able to find a manufacturer's OEL for atenolol.

Surface Contamination with Lactose

The surface levels of lactose are presented in Table 7; they ranged from ND (below the limit of detection of 0.0001 micrograms per square centimeter [µg/cm²]) to 19 µg/cm². Figure 6 shows the locations where the surface samples were collected. The highest contamination level was measured from a surface used in refilling canisters before it was cleaned; therefore, it should be considered a positive control. Lactose contamination varied throughout the pharmacy, but in general, higher amounts of lactose were found on work surfaces than on undisturbed areas (e.g., elevated shelving).

Table 7. Levels of lactose on surfaces during visit 2

Day	Location description	Sample no.*	Lactose ($\mu g/cm^2$)
1	Top shelf of Optifill workstation (7 feet high)	S1	0.0026
	Optifill workstation, in front of computer keyboard, next to fan	S2	0.040
	On top of Optifill machine, southwest corner (7 feet high)	S3	ND
	On top of Optifill machine, northeast corner (7 feet high)	S4	0.0005
	Shelf north of the Optifill machine	S5	ND
	Shelf in the Captain's office just to the left of the door (7 feet high)	S6	ND
	Top of shelf in vault area (7 feet high)	S7	0.0008
	Work surface in vault area	S8	0.32
	Aisle #4 top shelf (7 feet high)	S9	ND
	Corner of manual filling area (7 feet high)	S10	0.0008
	Shelf north of the Optifill machine where employee 21 was filling canisters	S11	19
	Computer mouse at Optifill workstation, next to fan	S12	0.056
2	On top of lockers in the break room	S13	0.065
	Prescription check workstation	S14	0.036
	Packaging workstation	S15	0.096
	PharmAssist computer #2 workstation	S16	0.30
	Manual fill station #2 computer mouse	S17	0.30
	Shelf above manual fill station #2 (8 feet high)	S18	0.056
Limit of detection			0.0001
Limit of quantitation			0.0003

*Sample numbers are provided for referring to sample locations in Figure 6.

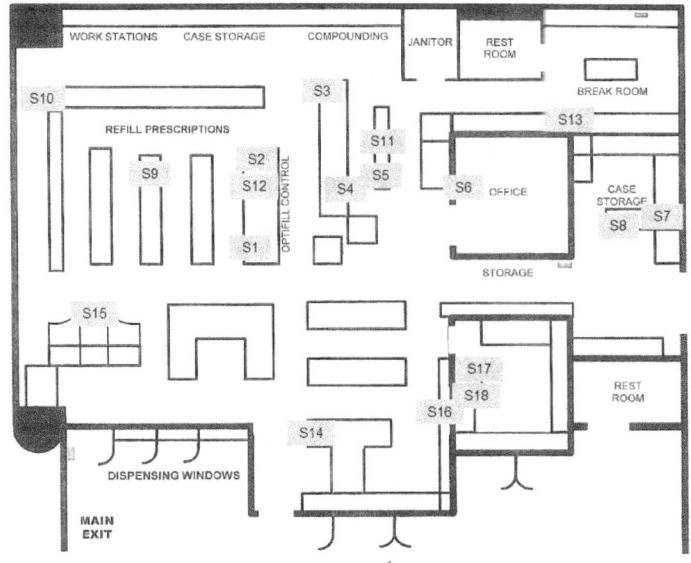

Figure 6. Surface sample locations during visit 2.

Use of Personal Protective Equipment and Other Observations

We observed sporadic use of nitrile gloves for all processes, and none of the employees wore protective clothing, eye protection, or respiratory protection during our visits. The vacuum was the only engineering control that was used, primarily for cleaning the Optifill machine. The Optifill machine was routinely cleaned once per day, and the vacuum filter was routinely changed every 3 to 4 months. We did not carefully monitor hand-washing activities before breaks.

Discussion

Several tasks involving uncoated tablets correlated with peaks in real-time particle number concentration and particle mass concentration. The largest increase in total particle number concentration occurred when canisters were cleaned using compressed air. Most of the particles released during cleaning with compressed air were < 3 µm in aerodynamic diameter. In comparison, during a previous evaluation at a large mail order pharmacy, particles > 10 µm in aerodynamic diameter contributed more to the total particle number concentrations measured during the cleaning of canisters without the use of compressed air. The maximum total particle number concentration measured during the cleaning of canisters in that evaluation was five times lower than in this evaluation [NIOSH 2011]. Therefore, the use of compressed air to clean canisters appears to generate higher particle number concentrations that are dominated by smaller particles (i.e., < 3 µm). These small particles have relatively slow settling velocities, meaning they can remain buoyant in air for hours, and they are capable of penetrating deep into the lungs. The slow settling velocities probably explains why we found elevated concentrations of particles with aerodynamic diameters < 1 µm more than 60 minutes after canisters had been cleaned with compressed air.

The use of the vacuum to clean the Optifill machine also produced elevated airborne particle number concentrations and personal inhalable dust concentrations (2,000 µg/m³) during that task. However, the particle number concentrations were dominated by submicron (< 1 µm) particles. Particles with an aerodynamic diameter around 0.3 µm are the most difficult to capture with filters [EPA 2008]. HEPA filters are required to have at least 99.97% collection efficiency for these particles [EPA 2008]. Therefore, using a HEPA-certified filter in the vacuum would likely reduce airborne levels of these small particles.

We measured personal air concentrations of total dust during visit 1 and inhalable dust during visit 2. Both of these sample types estimate what could be inhaled and deposited anywhere in the respiratory system [Kenny 1997; ACGIH 2012]. However, compared to inhalable dust samplers, total dust samplers can undersample particles > 30 µm in aerodynamic diameter [Kenny 1997]. These large particles are most likely to be deposited in the nose or mouth [Hinds 1999]. Because many APIs are water soluble, they can be absorbed in the upper respiratory system including nasal passages. Thus, inhalable dust is the most appropriate sample type for measuring exposure to pharmaceuticals. Lactose and specific APIs were analyzed on the inhalable dust samples (after the sample was weighed) but not the total dust samples.

The highest personal air concentrations of lactose, lisinopril, and HCTZ (inhalable dust) on visit 2 were measured on the employee who used compressed air to clean canisters. Two personal air concentrations of lisinopril measured on this employee were near or above the manufacturer's OEL of 1 µg/m³. This employee's side-by-side air sampling results varied by less than a factor of two. Although the DataRAM and Tygon tubing caused some of the total dust samples to underestimate the actual concentrations, the highest air concentrations of total dust on visit 1 were also measured on the employee who used compressed air to clean canisters. The total dust, inhalable dust, and lactose concentrations we measured are comparable to what we measured in a previous evaluation at a large mail order pharmacy. However, the personal air concentrations of lisinopril are higher than what we measured in that evaluation [NIOSH 2011].

In general, the highest area air concentrations of lisinopril and lactose were found near the Optifill machine where much of the compressed-air cleaning took place. Hard-to-reach surfaces had the lowest levels of lactose, and work surfaces used when directly handing APIs had the highest levels. This suggests that pharmaceutical dust was spread to many areas in the pharmacy, but was most concentrated near the areas where APIs were directly handled or canisters were cleaned using compressed air.

Most APIs do not have OELs set by federal agencies or national organizations. Because pharmaceuticals are biologically active and typically water soluble, OELs for nuisance dusts or "particles not otherwise specified" do not apply [ACGIH 2012]. Thus, we used manufacturers' OELs for comparing our results. Other than lisinopril, none of the measured APIs that had manufacturers' OELs were present in air at concentrations above their OELs. Possible acute health effects from high exposures to lisinopril listed on the safety data sheet included dizziness, headache, and allergic reactions [Bristol-Myers Squibb Company 2012b]. Maintaining airborne lisinopril exposures below the manufacturer's OEL should prevent these health effects in most employees. Although exposures to levothyroxine were below the manufacturer's OEL, the safety data sheet specifically recommends that, "All operations should be fully enclosed. No air recirculation permitted [Pfizer 2011]."

OELs typically do not consider possible synergistic effects from multiple API exposures. Although we could not measure all APIs in air, the nature of the work activities and the data we collected indicate that some employees were exposed to multiple APIs. The potential health effects from exposures to multiple APIs are largely unknown. Therefore, exposures to multiple APIs could present an unacceptable health risk to an employee, even if each individual API air concentration was below its manufacturer's OEL.

In addition to the inhalation route, pharmaceuticals that deposit onto unprotected skin and are not washed off could be inadvertently ingested. Some pharmaceuticals, depending on their chemical makeup, could also be absorbed through the skin. Unprotected eyes could also be a route of absorption for pharmaceuticals. Finally, pharmaceuticals on personal clothing could be brought home and potentially be a source of exposure for family members. Children may be especially susceptible to adverse health effects from API exposures [Brent et al. 2004]. These routes of exposure are pertinent at this workplace as nitrile gloves were used sporadically, and protective clothing and safety glasses were not used at all during our visits.

Conclusions

Use of compressed air to clean automatic dispensing machine canisters caused the largest releases of dust. Uncoated tablets were the main source of this dust. Although we did not quantify all possible APIs in air, multiple APIs were detected in employees' personal breathing zones. For the APIs with exposure criteria, most air concentrations (except for one personal air concentration of lisinopril) were below the manufacturers' OELs. However, OELs do not consider possible synergistic effects from multiple API exposures. Lactose, an inactive filler in tablets, was present on work surfaces, suggesting that surface contamination with APIs was also possible. Recommendations are listed below to reduce pharmaceutical dust exposures. Eliminating the use of compressed air, in particular, should substantially reduce airborne exposures and surface contamination levels of pharmaceuticals.

Recommendations

We encourage the pharmacy to use a labor-management health and safety committee or working group to discuss the recommendations in this report and develop an action plan. These recommendations are based on the hierarchy of controls approach that groups actions by their likely effectiveness in reducing or removing hazards.

An important first step in the management of occupational exposures to pharmaceuticals is obtaining information on the potential for workplace exposures to APIs and risk of those exposures. We gathered some of this information during our evaluation. However, additional information should be gathered now and in the future, especially as new pharmaceuticals and formulations enter the market. We recommend determining which pharmaceuticals are dusty. Although uncoated tablets are generally dusty, employees may be able to identify those that produce more dust. We also recommend obtaining safety data sheets and reviewing manufacturer exposure guidelines and toxicity data for all tablets. Safety data sheets from the original manufacturer of the name-brand pharmaceutical may contain the most detailed information. This information can then be used to develop a priority list of dusty pharmaceuticals that are potentially hazardous at low concentrations (e.g., manufacturers' OELs < 10 $\mu g/m^3$). Employees who handle these pharmaceuticals in ways that could cause the dust to become airborne may require a higher level of protection.

Engineering Controls

Engineering controls reduce employees' exposures by removing the hazard from the process or by placing a barrier between the hazard and the employee. Engineering controls protect employees effectively without placing primary responsibility of implementation on the employee.

1. Install a partially enclosed local exhaust hood that is ducted outdoors. Use this hood when filling prescriptions or refilling canisters with pharmaceuticals on your priority list. Ducting the hood outdoors will prevent the re-entrainment of APIs into the work environment. For some APIs (e.g., levothyroxine), the manufacturer specifically states that no air recirculation is permitted. The American Conference of Governmental Industrial Hygienists Industrial Ventilation Manual provides guidelines on the optimal duct and face velocity for the control of very fine light dusts [ACGIH 2010].

2. Use a HEPA vacuum with a long narrow tip to clean hard to reach areas of the automatic dispensing machine canisters rather than using compressed air to clean the canisters. Make sure the filter in the vacuum is HEPA certified and properly seated in the vacuum. Doing this process inside the local exhaust hood would help further control small particles that penetrate the HEPA filter or are otherwise generated by the cleaning process. Disconnect the compressed air line if it has no other purpose.

Administrative Controls

The term "administrative controls" refers to employer-dictated work practices and policies to reduce or prevent hazardous exposures. Their effectiveness depends on employer commitment and employee acceptance. Regular monitoring and reinforcement are necessary to ensure that policies and procedures are followed consistently.

1. Consult a ventilation specialist to install and commission the local exhaust hood. Hood performance should be validated at least annually.

2. Train employees annually on how to properly use and maintain the local exhaust hood.

3. Replace the HEPA vacuum filter cartridge according to the manufacturer's guidelines. Wear nitrile gloves and work under the hood when performing this task.

4. Use the HEPA vacuum daily to clean the Optifill machine and collect pharmaceutical dust that accumulates under the canisters. Wear nitrile gloves, long-sleeve protective clothing, and safety glasses when performing this task.

5. Clean any residual dust on work surfaces with isopropyl alcohol wipes before breaks and at the end of the day. Wear nitrile gloves when cleaning surfaces.

6. Remind employees of the importance of washing their hands before eating or using tobacco products to prevent the hand-to-mouth ingestion of pharmaceutical particles.

Personal Protective Equipment

Personal protective equipment is the least effective means for controlling hazardous exposures. Proper use of personal protective equipment requires a comprehensive program and a high level of employee involvement and commitment. The right personal protective equipment must be chosen for each hazard. Supporting programs such as training, change-out schedules, and medical assessment may be needed. Personal protective equipment should not be the sole method for controlling hazardous exposures. Rather, personal protective equipment should be used until effective engineering and administrative controls are in place.

1. Train employees on the importance of wearing nitrile gloves when handling pharmaceuticals, working with objects containing pharmaceutical dust, or cleaning surfaces with pharmaceutical dust.

2. Provide safety glasses and long-sleeve protective clothing to employees who perform tasks outside the hood that could generate airborne pharmaceutical dust. The protective clothing should either be disposable or kept at work and laundered weekly by a laundry service. Wearing protective clothing should minimize the potential for take home exposure.

Appendix A: Additional Information on Pharmaceutical Analytical Methods

Gravimetric analysis of the personal and area air samples was performed using NIOSH Methods 0500 and 0600 [NIOSH 2012]. After gravimetric analysis, the air samples were further analyzed for lactose and/or specific APIs using BVNA methods. The surface wipe samples were also analyzed for lactose using a BVNA method. These methods are briefly summarized below for each analyte.

Lactose

Filters were removed from the IOM samplers and extracted in glass vials using 2 milliliters (mL) of deionized water and sonicated for 15 minutes. After extraction, the samples were transferred to autosampler vials and analyzed by high performance liquid chromatography using the parameters below.

> Instrument: Dionex 3000
> Column: Dionex CarboPac PA1, 4 x 250 mm
> Column flow rate: 1 mL per minute
> Column temperature: Ambient
> Injection volume: 200 microliter
> Detector: Electrochemical detector
> Mobile phase: Isocratic, 200 millimolar (mM) sodium hydroxide in deionized water

Lisinopril and Hydrochlorothiazide

Filters were processed as described for lactose analysis and analyzed by high performance liquid chromatography using the parameters below.

> Instrument: Agilent 1100
> Column: Waters Spherisorb C8, 150 mm x 4.6 mm 5 μm particle size
> Column flow rate: 1 mL per minute
> Column temperature: 40°C
> Injection volume: 30 microliter
> Detector: Ultraviolet/visible
> Wavelength: 215 nanometer
> Mobile phase: Isocratic 85% (Dipotassium phosphate, 0.1% phosphoric acid)/15% methanol

Loratadine

Filters were desorbed in 2 mL of a 40% (1% triethylamine, 0.75% phosphoric acid)/60% acetonitrile solution and sonicated for 15 minutes. Samples were transferred to autosampler vials for analysis by high performance liquid chromatography using the parameters below.

> Instrument: Dionex ICS 3000
> Column: Dionex CarboPac PA1, 250 mm by 4 mm
> Column flow rate: 1 mL per minute
> Column temperature: Ambient
> Injection volume: 200 microliter
> Detector: Ultraviolet/visible
> Wavelength: 215 nanometer
> Mobile phase: Isocratic 40% (1% triethylamine, 0.75% phosphoric acid)/60% acetonitrile

Hydrocodone, Oxycodone, and Codeine

Filters were desorbed in 2 mL of a 50% (15 mM sodium lauryl sulfate, 15 mM dipotassium phosphate, 0.1% phosphoric acid)/5% acetonitrile/45% methanol solution and sonicated for 15 minutes. Samples were transferred to autosampler vials for analysis by high performance liquid chromatography using the parameters below.

    Instrument: Agilent 1100
    Column: MacMod Halo C18, 4.6 mm by 75 mm, 2.7 μm particle size
    Column flow rate: 1.5 mL per minute
    Column temperature: 40°C
    Injection volume: 50 microliter
    Detector: Ultraviolet/visible
    Wavelength: 210 nanometer
    Mobile phase: Isocratic 50% 15 mM sodium lauryl sulfate, 15 mM dipotassium phosphate, 0.1% phosphoric acid, 5% acetonitrile

Atenolol

Filters were desorbed in 2 mL of a 92.5% 100 mM dipotassium phosphate/7.5% acetonitrile solution and sonicated for 15 minutes. Samples were transferred to autosampler vials for analysis by high performance liquid chromatography using the parameters below.

    Instrument: Agilent 1100
    Column: Xterrra C18, 150 mm by 4.6 mm, 3.5 μm particle size
    Column flow rate: 1 mL per minute
    Column temperature: Ambient
    Injection volume: 50 microliter
    Detector: Ultraviolet/visible
    Wavelength: 226 nanometer
    Mobile phase: Isocratic 92.5% 100 mM dipotassium phosphate/7.5% acetonitrile

Levothyroxine

Filters were desorbed in 20 nanogram/mL thyroxine in 30% deionized water (0.1% formic acid)/70% acetonitrile solution and sonicated for 15 minutes. Samples were transferred to autosampler vials for analysis by liquid chromatography/tandem mass spectrometry using the parameters below.

    Instrument: Agilent 1100
    Column: Atlantis Hilic Silica, 50 mm by 2.1 mm, 3 μm pore size
    Column flow rate: 0.3 mL per minute
    Column temperature: 35°C
    Injection volume: 20 microliter
    Detector: AB Sciex API 3000 MS/MS with turbo ion spry source
    Source temperature: 350°C
    MS function: Multiple reaction monitoring
    Levothyroxine quantitation transition: 777.8–731.8 atomic mass units
    Thyroxine (internal standard) transition: 783.78–737.65 atomic mass units
    Mobile phase: Isocratic 30% deionized water (0.1% formic acid)/70% acetonitrile (0.1% formic acid)

Appendix B: Real-Time Particle Measurement Results

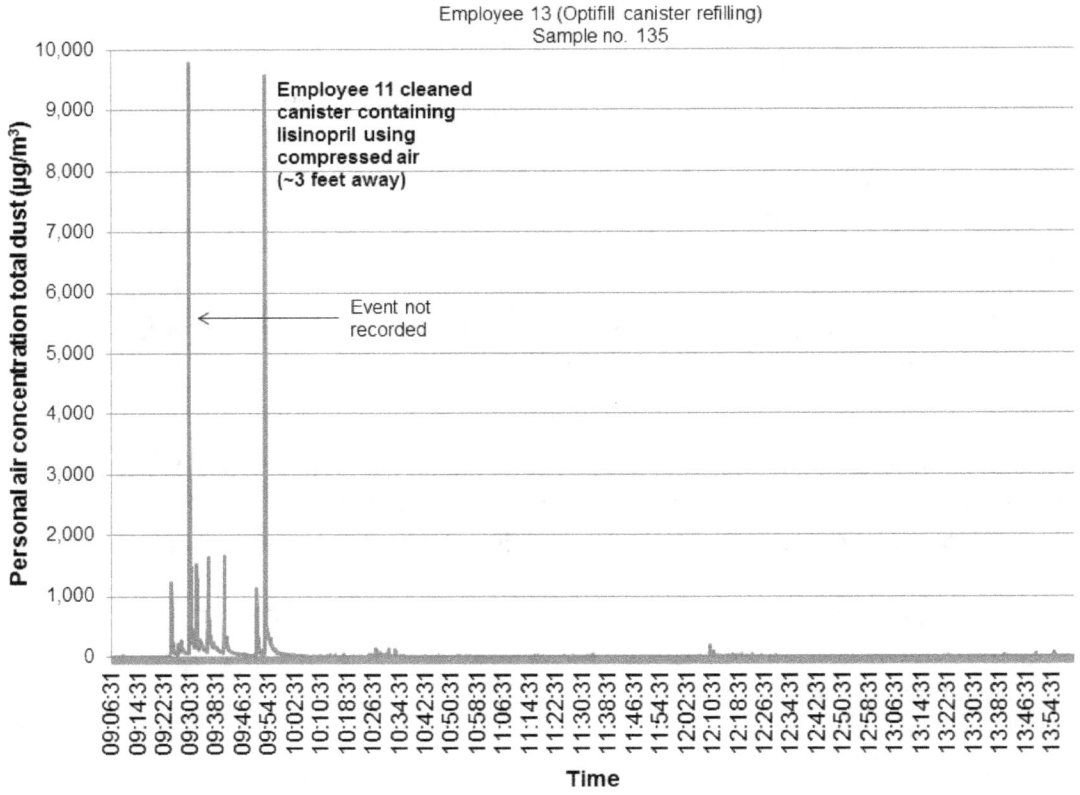

Figure B1. Real-time mass concentration of total dust measured in the personal breathing zone of employee 13 who refilled Optifill canisters during day 1 of visit 1. Tasks associated with increases in mass concentrations are noted in the figure.

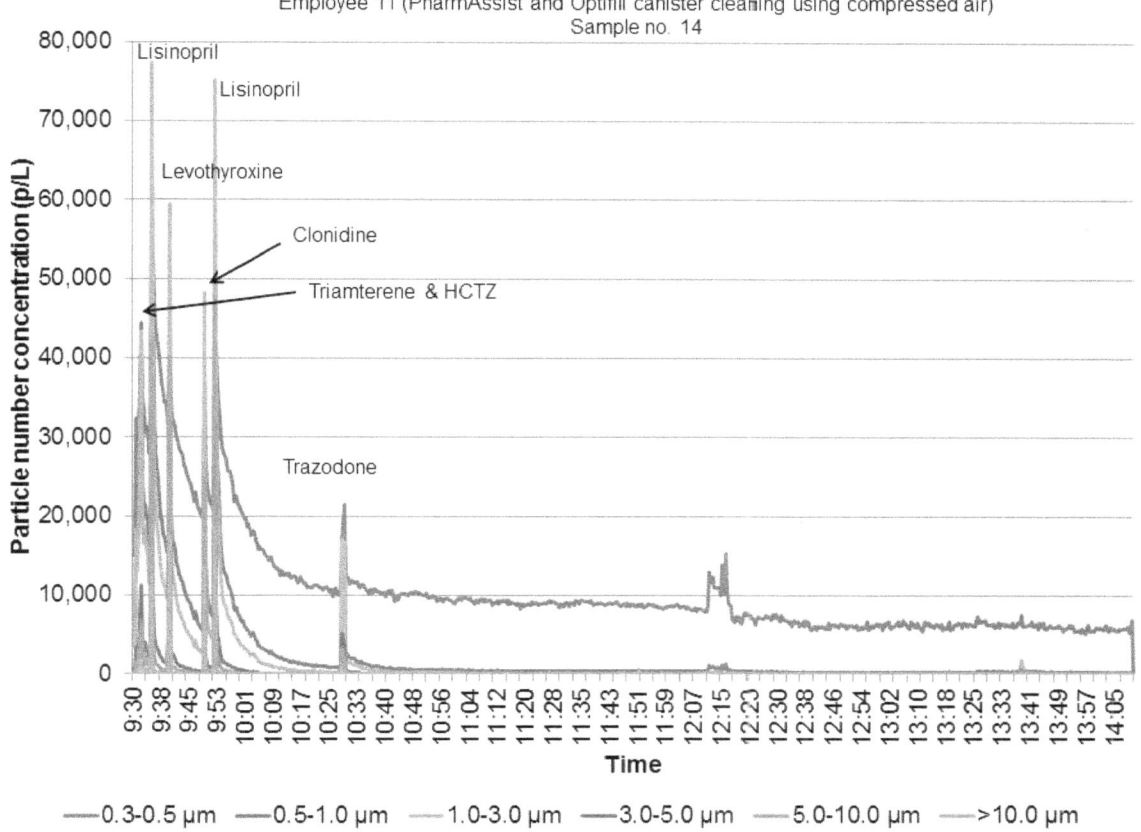

Figure B2. Real-time particle number concentrations measured near the personal breathing zone of employee 11 who cleaned canisters using compressed air during day 1 of visit 1. The APIs contained in the canisters that were cleaned are noted above the peaks in particle concentrations that occurred at the same time.

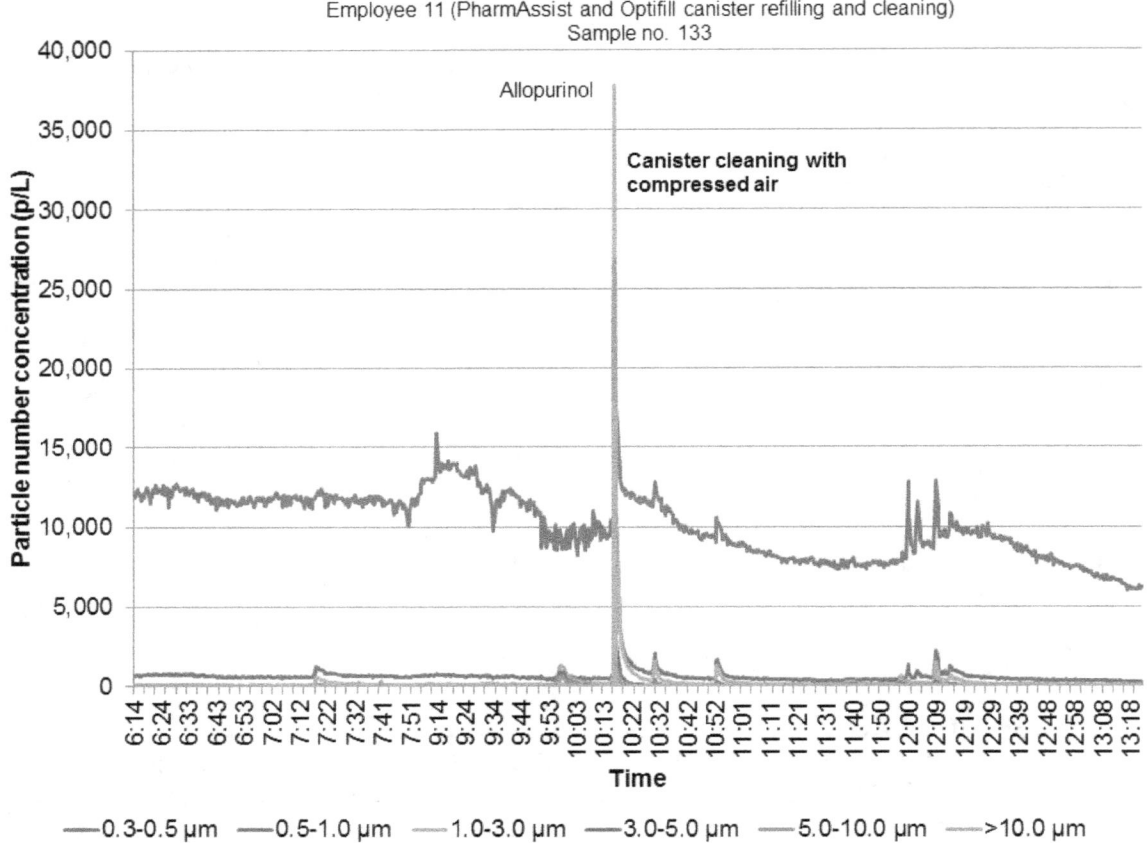

Figure B3. Real-time particle number concentrations measured near the personal breathing zone of employee 11 who refilled and cleaned canisters using compressed air during day 2 of visit 1. The APIs contained in the canisters that were cleaned are noted above the peaks in particle concentrations that occurred at the same time.

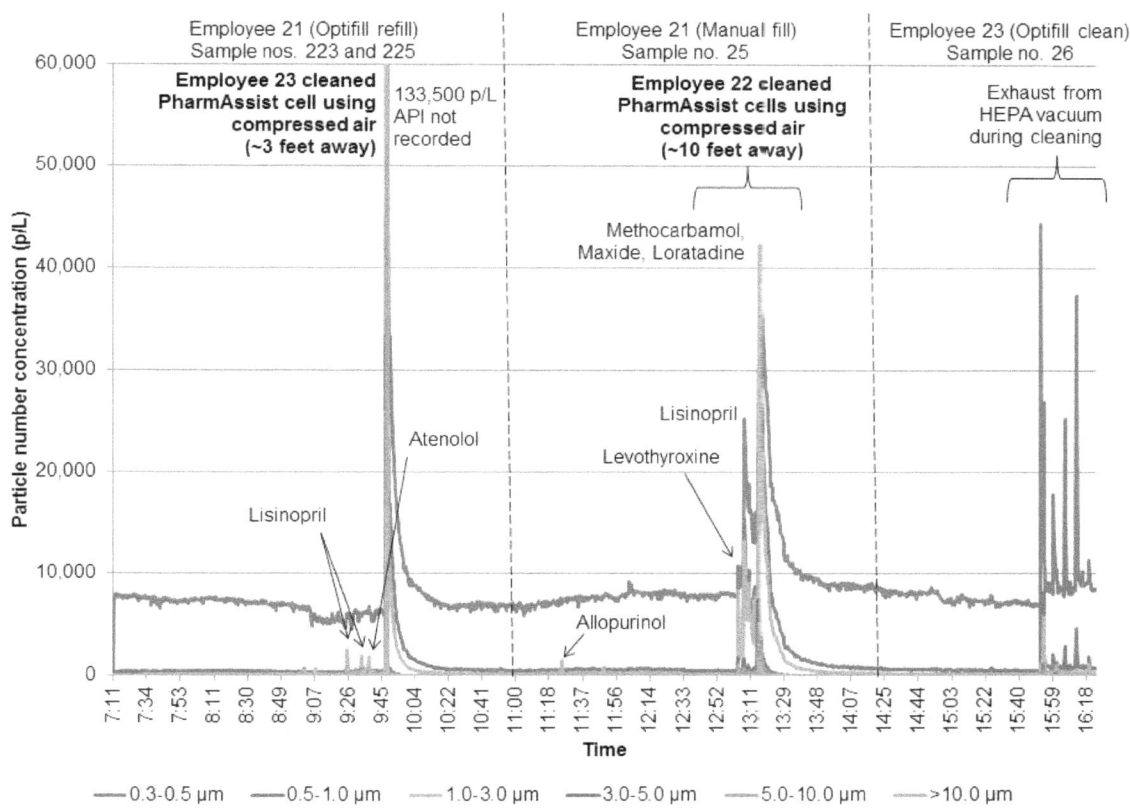

Figure B4. Real-time particle number concentrations measured near the personal breathing zones of employee 21 (who performed Optifill refill during the first part of the day and manual fill during the second part of the day) and employee 26 (who cleaned the Optifil machine towards the end of the day) during day 1 of visit 2. The APIs that were handled during these tasks are noted above the peaks in particle concentrations that occurred at the same time. The largest increases in particle concentrations were due to tasks performed by nearby employees, which are also noted above the corresponding peaks.

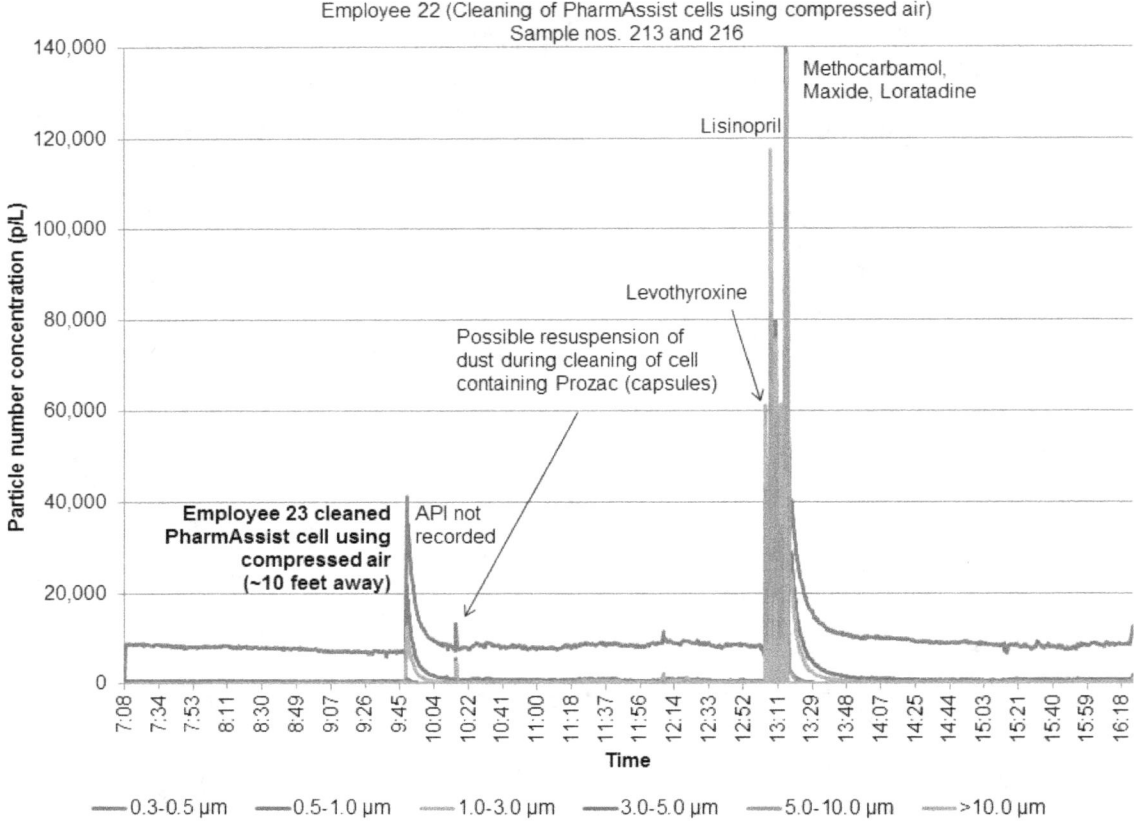

Figure B5. Real-time particle concentrations measured near the personal breathing zone of employee 22, who used compressed air to clean PharmAssist canisters during day 1 of visit 2. The APIs contained in the canisters that were cleaned are noted above the peaks in particle concentrations that occurred at the same time. Other tasks performed by nearby employees that also resulted in increased particle concentrations are noted above the corresponding peaks.

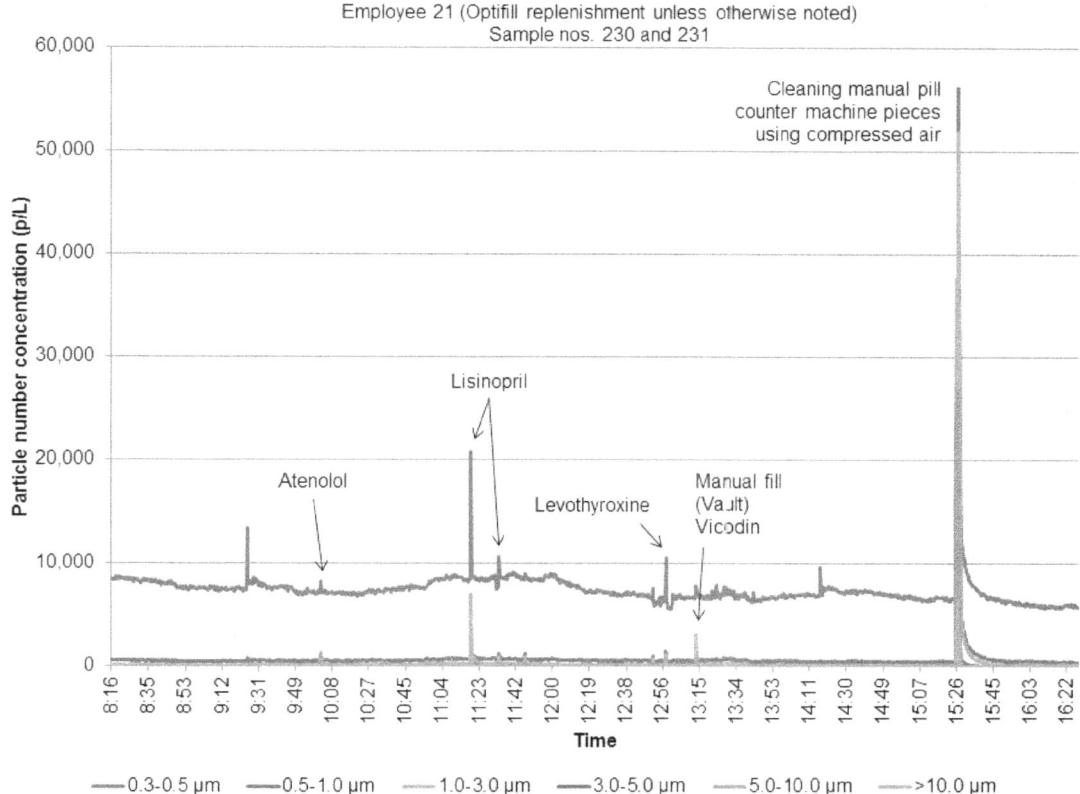

Figure B6. Real-time particle number concentrations measured near the personal breathing zone of employee 21, who mostly performed Optifill refill during day 2 of visit 2. The APIs that were handled during refill are noted above the peaks in particle concentrations that occurred at the same time. Cleaning of the manual pill counter machine, which resulted in the largest increase in particle concentration, is also noted above the corresponding peak.

Appendix C: Occupational Exposure Limits and Health Effects

NIOSH investigators refer to mandatory (legally enforceable) and recommended OELs for chemical, physical, and biological agents when evaluating workplace hazards. OELs have been developed by federal agencies and safety and health organizations to prevent adverse health effects from workplace exposures. Generally, OELs suggest levels of exposure that most employees may be exposed to for up to 10 hours per day, 40 hours per week, for a working lifetime, without experiencing adverse health effects. However, not all employees will be protected if their exposures are maintained below these levels. Some may have adverse health effects because of individual susceptibility, a pre-existing medical condition, or a hypersensitivity (allergy). In addition, some hazardous substances act in combination with other exposures, with the general environment, or with medications or personal habits of the employee to produce adverse health effects. Most OELs address airborne exposures, but some substances can be absorbed directly through the skin and mucous membranes.

Most OELs are expressed as a TWA exposure. A TWA refers to the average exposure during a normal 8- to 10-hour workday. Some chemical substances and physical agents have recommended short-term exposure limits or ceiling values. Unless otherwise noted, the short-term exposure limit is a 15-minute TWA exposure. It should not be exceeded at any time during a workday. The ceiling limit should not be exceeded at any time.

In the United States, OELs have been established by federal agencies, professional organizations, state and local governments, and other entities. Some OELs are legally enforceable limits; others are recommendations.

- The U.S. Department of Labor Occupational Safety and Health Administration permissible exposure limits (29 CFR 1910 [general industry]; 29 CFR 1926 [construction industry]; and 29 CFR 1917 [maritime industry]) are legal limits. These limits are enforceable in workplaces covered under the Occupational Safety and Health Act of 1970.

- NIOSH recommended exposure limits are recommendations based on a critical review of the scientific and technical information and the adequacy of methods to identify and control the hazard. NIOSH recommended exposure limits are published in the *NIOSH Pocket Guide to Chemical Hazards* [NIOSH 2010]. NIOSH also recommends risk management practices (e.g., engineering controls, safe work practices, employee education/training, personal protective equipment, and exposure and medical monitoring) to minimize the risk of exposure and adverse health effects.

- Other OELs commonly used and cited in the United States include the Threshold Limit Values, which are recommended by the American Conference of Governmental Industrial Hygienists, a professional organization, and the workplace environmental exposure levels, which are recommended by the American Industrial Hygiene Association, another professional organization. The Threshold Limit Values and workplace environmental exposure levels are developed by committee members of these associations from a review of the published, peer-reviewed literature. These OELs are not consensus standards. Threshold Limit Values are considered voluntary exposure guidelines for use by industrial hygienists and others trained in this discipline "to assist in the control of health hazards" [ACGIH 2012]. Workplace environmental exposure levels have been established for some chemicals "when no other legal or authoritative limits exist" [AIHA 2011].

Outside the United States, OELs have been established by various agencies and organizations and include legal and recommended limits. The Institut für Arbeitsschutz der Deutschen Gesetzlichen Unfallversicherung (Institute for Occupational Safety and Health of the German Social Accident Insurance) maintains a database of international OELs from European Union member states, Canada (Québec), Japan, Switzerland, and the United States. The database, available at http://www.dguv.de/ifa/en/gestis/limit_values/index.jsp, contains international limits for more than 1,500 hazardous substances and is updated periodically.

The Occupational Safety and Health Administration requires an employer to furnish employees a place of employment free from recognized hazards that cause or are likely to cause death or serious physical harm [Occupational Safety and Health Act of 1970 (Public Law 91–596, sec. 5(a)(1))]. This is true in the absence of a specific OEL. It also is important to keep in mind that OELs may not reflect current health-based information.

When multiple OELs exist for a substance or agent, NIOSH investigators generally encourage employers to use the lowest OEL when making risk assessment and risk management decisions. NIOSH investigators also encourage use of the hierarchy of controls approach to eliminate or minimize workplace hazards. This includes, in order of preference, the use of (1) substitution or elimination of the hazardous agent, (2) engineering controls (e.g., local exhaust ventilation, process enclosure, dilution ventilation), (3) administrative controls (e.g., limiting time of exposure, employee training, work practice changes, medical surveillance), and (4) personal protective equipment (e.g., respiratory protection, gloves, eye protection, hearing protection).

Active Pharmaceutical Ingredients

None of the APIs measured in air have OELs established by federal agencies or national organizations. However, many of them do have OELs established by pharmaceutical companies using a control banding process. Control banding, a qualitative risk assessment and risk management tool, is a complementary approach to protecting employee health that focuses resources on exposure controls by describing how a risk needs to be managed. This approach can be applied in situations where authoritative OELs have not been established or can be used to supplement such OELs. In the pharmaceutical industry, APIs are placed into hazard categories using data such as potency, severity of acute effects, lethal dose, irritation, and sensitization [Naumann et al. 1996; Naumann 2005; Zalk and Nelson 2008]. Once placed into hazard categories, pharmaceuticals are often assigned OELs or hazard control bands. Pharmaceutical companies may provide these OELs or hazard control bands on their safety data sheets, along with potential acute and chronic health effects from workplace exposures. Table C1 provides the manufacturers' OELs or hazard control bands for the APIs measured in this evaluation. Other manufacturers may have OELs in addition to those listed in Table C1. Maintaining exposures below these manufacturers' OELs should minimize any potential health effects. However, OELs typically do not consider possible synergistic effects from multiple API exposures. More information on control banding is available at http://www.cdc.gov/niosh/topics/ctrlbanding/.

Table C1. Prescribed uses and manufacturers' TWA-OELs for the APIs measured in air

API	Prescribed for*	Manufacturer's OEL or hazard control band ($\mu g/m^3$)†
Atenolol	High blood pressure	None published
Codeine	Pain relief or cough suppression	100
HCTZ	High blood pressure and fluid retention	100
Hydrocodone	Pain relief or cough suppression	5
Lisinopril	High blood pressure, heart failure	1–10
Loratadine	Allergies	None published
Oxycodone	Pain relief	40
Levothyroxine	Hypothyroidism	< 1

*[PubMed Health 2012]

†Codeine [GlaxoSmithKline 2006], HCTZ [Bristol-Myers Squibb Company 2012a], Hydrocodone [Abbott Labs 2011], Lisinopril [Bristol-Myers Squibb Company 2012b], Oxycodone [Purdue Pharma LP 2008], Levothyroxine [Pfizer 2011].

References

Abbott Labs [2011]. Safety data sheet: Vicodin ES tablets. [http://www.abbott.com/global/url/content/en_US/20.40:40/general_content/General_Content_00183.htm]. Date accessed: April 2013.

ACGIH [2010]. Industrial ventilation: a manual of recommended practice for design, 27th edition. Cincinnati, OH: American Conference of Governmental Industrial Hygienists.

ACGIH [2012]. Threshold limit values for chemical substances and physical agents and biological exposure indices. Cincinnati, OH: American Conference of Governmental Industrial Hygienists.

AIHA [2011]. AIHA 2012 Emergency response planning guidelines (ERPG) & workplace environmental exposure levels (WEEL) handbook. Fairfax, VA: American Industrial Hygiene Association.

Brent RL, Tanski S, Weitzman M [2004]. A pediatric perspective on the unique vulnerability and resilience of the embryo and the child to environmental toxicants: the importance of rigorous research concerning age and agent. Pediatrics *113*(4 Suppl):935–944.

Bristol-Myers Squibb Company [2012a]. Safety data sheet: Hydrochlorothiazide. [http://www.bmsmsds.com/msdsweb/]. Date accessed: April 2013.

Bristol-Myers Squibb Company [2012b]. Safety data sheet: Lisinopril. [http://www.bmsmsds.com/msdsweb/]. Date accessed: April 2013.

CFR. Code of Federal Regulations. Washington, DC: U.S. Government Printing Office, Office of the Federal Register.

EPA [2008]. Residential air cleaners (second edition): a summary of available information. Washington, DC; U.S. Environmental Protection Agency, Office of Air and Radiation, Indoor Environment Division. Publication No. EPA 402-F-09-002. [http://www.epa.gov/iaq/pdfs/residential_air_cleaners.pdf]. Date accessed: April 2013.

GlaxoSmithKline [2006]. Safety data sheet: Solpadeine plus soluble tablets. [http://www.msds-gsk.com/uk_cons/0022200b.pdf]. Date accessed: April 2013.

Hinds WC [1999]. Respiratory deposition. In: Aerosol technology: properties, behavior, and measurement of airborne particles. New York: John Wiley & Sons, Inc.

Kenny LC, Aitken R, Chalmers C, Fabries JF, Gonzalez-Fernandez E, Kromhout H, Liden G, Mark D, Riediger G, Prodi V [1997]. A collaborative European study of personal inhalable aerosol sampler performance. Ann Occup Hyg *41*(2):135–153.

Naumann BD [2005]. Control banding in the pharmaceutical industry. [http://www.aioh.org.au/downloads/documents/ControlBandingBNaumann.pdf]. Date accessed: April 2013.

Naumann BD, Sargent EV, Starkman BS, Fraser WJ, Becker GT, Kirk GD [1996]. Performance-based exposure control limits for pharmaceutical active ingredients. Am Ind Hyg Assoc J 57(1):33–42.

NIOSH [2010]. NIOSH pocket guide to chemical hazards. Cincinnati, OH: U.S. Department of Health and Human Services, Centers for Disease Control and Prevention, National Institute for Occupational Safety and Health (NIOSH) Publication No. 2010-168c. [http://www.cdc.gov/niosh/npg/]. Date accessed: April 2013.

NIOSH [2011]. Health hazard evaluation report: exposures to pharmaceutical dust at a mail order pharmacy – Illinois. By Fent KW, Durgam S, Aristeguieta C, Brueck SE. Cincinnati, OH: U.S. Department of Health and Human Services, Centers for Disease Control and Prevention, National Institute for Occupational Safety and Health, NIOSH HETA No. 2010-0026-3150.

NIOSH [2012]. NIOSH manual of analytical methods. 4th ed. Schlecht PC, O'Connor PF, eds. Cincinnati, OH: U.S. Department of Health and Human Services, Centers for Disease Control and Prevention, National Institute for Occupational Safety and Health, DHHS (NIOSH) Publication No. 94-113 (August 1994); 1st Supplement Publication 96-135, 2nd Supplement Publication 98-119, 3rd Supplement Publication 2003-154. [http://www.cdc.gov/niosh/docs/2003-154/].

Pfizer [2011]. Safety data sheet: Levothyroxine sodium tablets. [http://www.pfizer.com/files/products/material_safety_data/PZ01680.pdf]. Date accessed: April 2013.

Purdue Pharma L.P. [2008]. Material safety data sheet: OxyContin tablets. [http://www.purduepharma.com/msdss/Oxycontin_Binder.pdf]. Date accessed: April 2013.

PubMed Health [2012]. Drugs and supplements. [http://www.ncbi.nlm.nih.gov/pubmedhealth/s/drugs_and_supplements/a/]. Date accessed: April 2013.

Thermo [1995]. Thermo technical guidelines: inlet tubing guidelines for MIE dust monitors. Franklin, MA: Thermo Electron Corporation Publication No. 19-A.

Zalk DM, Nelson DI [2008]. History and evolution of control banding: a review. J Occup Environ Hyg 5(5):330–346.

Keywords: NAICS 446110 (Pharmacies and Drug Stores), drugs, pills, pill dust, active pharmaceutical ingredients, APIs, tablets, pharmaceuticals, outpatient pharmacy, retail pharmacy, automatic pill dispensing machine, robotic pill dispenser

The Health Hazard Evaluation Program investigates possible health hazards in the workplace under the authority of Section 20(a)(6) of the Occupational Safety and Health Act of 1970, 29 U.S.C. 669(a)(6). The Health Hazard Evaluation Program also provides, upon request, technical assistance to federal, state, and local agencies to control occupational health hazards and to prevent occupational illness and disease. Regulations guiding the Program can be found in Title 42, Code of Federal Regulations, Part 85; Requests for Health Hazard Evaluations (42 CFR 85).

Acknowledgments

Analytical Support: Bureau Veritas North America
Desktop Publishers: Greg Hartle and Mary Winfree
Editor: Ellen Galloway
Health Communicator: Stefanie Brown
Logistics: Donnie Booher and Karl Feldmann

Availability of Report

Copies of this report have been sent to the employer, employees, and union at the facility. The state and local health department and the Occupational Safety and Health Administration Regional Office have also received a copy. This report is not copyrighted and may be freely reproduced.

This report is available at http://www.cdc.gov/niosh/hhe/reports/pdfs/2010-0078-3177.pdf

Recommended citation for this report:
NIOSH [2013]. Health hazard evaluation report: evaluation of pharmaceutical dust exposures at an outpatient pharmacy. By Fent KW, Durgam S*, Methner M. Cincinnati, OH: U.S. Department of Health and Human Services, Centers for Disease Control and Prevention, National Institute for Occupational Safety and Health, NIOSH HETA No. 2010-0078-3177.

*Currently with General Electric, Niskayuna, New York.

Delivering on the Nation's promise:
Safety and health at work for all people through research and prevention

To receive NIOSH documents or more information about occupational safety and health topics, please contact NIOSH:

Telephone: 1–800–CDC–INFO (1–800–232–4636)

TTY: 1–888–232–6348

CDC INFO: www.cdc.gov/info

or visit the NIOSH Web site at www.cdc.gov/niosh

For a monthly update on news at NIOSH, subscribe to NIOSH eNews by visiting www.cdc.gov/niosh/eNews.

SAFER • HEALTHIER • PEOPLE™